The 1993–1994 Debate on Health Care Reform

The 1993–1994 Debate on Health Care Reform

Did the Polls Mislead the Policy Makers?

Karlyn H. Bowman

The author wishes to thank Everett Carll Ladd, professor of political science and director of the Roper Center at the University of Connecticut, for his sage advice about American public opinion generally and for his willingness to review this monograph. Christine Doane and Jennifer Baggette provided invaluable assistance in preparing it.

The Henry J. Kaiser Family Foundation made the publication of this monograph possible. It is a sequel to *Public Attitudes on Health Care Reform: Are the Polls Misleading the Policy Makers?*

Contents

Introduction

In early October 1994, the Gallup Organization asked Americans how they felt about the fact that Congress had not passed a health care bill. A majority (53 percent) told the pollsters that they were "relieved," while 38 percent said that they were "angry." The results were not substantially different from those Gallup obtained when the organization first posed a similar question in August. Why would a population that seemed so supportive of health care reform a year earlier have come to this conclusion? And why would an issue that generated so much commentary as a potentially decisive election issue have "virtually vanished from the midterm campaign"? Those words, written by *Washington Post* columnist David Broder eleven days before the November election, summarized what most reporters found on the campaign trail.

Did the polls mislead the policy makers about the importance of this issue and the urgency of reform? This monograph is a response to that question, a review of the attitudinal data collected during the 1993–1994 debate on health care reform, and a look ahead at how future reforms could fare in the court of public opinion.

In the spring of 1994, I wrote a monograph for AEI entitled *Public Attitudes on Health Care Reform: Are the Polls Misleading the Policy Makers?* The study was designed to bring together survey data from polls in the public domain to help policy makers understand attitudes about the health care system and proposals for reforming it. I also looked at how the pollsters tackled the subject. I did not plan to revisit public attitudes, but the opportunity was provided unexpectedly by Drew Altman, president of the Henry J. Kaiser Family Foundation, who offered to support publication of a sequel to update the compilation of survey data. I am very grateful to Mr. Altman and the Kaiser Family Foundation for making it possible for me to take another look at one of the most intensely polled subjects in recent memory. Neither Mr. Altman nor the Kaiser Family Foundation had any editorial involvement in this study.

Policy makers could gain considerable insight into public thinking from the scores of questions that were asked about health care before and during the 1993–1994 debate; but they could also be misled. Profound continuities coexisted in the data with substantial ambiguity. As this is being written in early November 1994, the pollsters seem to have abandoned the subject of health care reform, an area they probed extensively in the fall of 1993 and in the winter, spring, and summer of 1994. Still, the vast collection of survey data they amassed on this subject during 1993 and 1994 will be a useful guide to public opinion on any future reform effort.

What the Polls Told Us

Polling carried out during the 1993–1994 debate on health care reform was generally responsible and informative, particularly in the first and second of four major waves of attitudinal research. The first wave of polls concentrated on deepening our understanding of how Americans assessed the current system. The second wave began after President Clinton announced his health care reform plan on September 22, 1993, and the pollsters attempted to probe attitudes toward the total effort. This wave provided much useful information about the concerns people had about reform.

The third wave of questions attempted to divine how much support existed for specific reform proposals. No matter how carefully these questions were worded—and many were impressive as descriptions of enormously complex policy proposals—the questions were virtually meaningless as a guide to action. Polls suggesting, for example, that Americans were opting for an employer mandate over a single-payer system or an individual mandate were attempts to provide certainty where none existed. The pollsters asked these questions in the face of substantial evidence that the public was not well informed about specific plans or possible consequences of their enactment. These questions, discussed in the section of this report titled "The Clinton Plan," did not illuminate the public's thinking. They were posed largely because polls that continued to mine familiar ground no longer made headlines. In the highly competitive business that survey research has become, pollsters were going beyond areas where opinion could be useful to policy makers. The fourth wave of polling attempted to measure the political consequences for the November 1994 elections of a legislator's vote for or against a health care reform proposal. These questions are a familiar fixture of polling these days, but they are also of limited value.

The Current System

Louis Harris and Associates have been asking Americans for the past decade to select among three viewpoints about the performance of the health care system. The question not only provides a current measure of opinion but also allows us to see how attitudes have changed over time. Harris's first option is as follows: on the whole, the health care system works pretty well and only minor changes are necessary to make it work better. The second option is stated this way: there are some good things in our health care system, but fundamental changes are needed to make it better. The third response category is as follows: our health care system has so much wrong with it that we need to rebuild it completely.

Those saying the health care system works pretty well and needs only minor changes have been in the minority in all nine iterations of this question over the past decade. In 1982, only 19 percent felt that way; in 1994, 14 percent did. In 1982, 28 percent said that the system needed to be completely rebuilt. By 1994 that percentage had edged up to 31 percent. A plurality in 1982 (47 percent) and a majority in 1994 (54 percent) said that there are good things about the system but that fundamental changes are needed to make it better (see table 1). A very similar CBS News/*New York Times* question asked in September 1994 produced virtually identical results. Nineteen percent said that only minor changes in the system were needed, 31 percent said that the system needed to be completely rebuilt, and 48 percent said that "there are some good things in our health care system, but fundamental changes are needed."

Questions about whether the system is in crisis made more compelling newspaper headlines and television sound bites during the debate than did the Harris or CBS News/*New York Times* questions, but they did not tell us much about how Americans evaluated their care or the current system. In a period of just twenty-six days, for example, 84 percent of Americans in one Gallup poll (for CNN and *USA Today*, January 15–17, 1994) said that "there is a health care crisis in this country," while only 43 percent expressed the same sentiment in another poll (Yankelovich Partners for *Time* and CNN, February 10, 1994). It is highly unlikely that the health care crisis diminished substantially in a month's time, of course. The questions were worded slightly differently, and that accounted in part for the dissimilar responses. But a more likely explanation is that the "crisis" formulation did not capture the way Americans thought about the health care system, and so answers shifted depending on slight changes in question wording or emphasis from poll to poll.

TABLE 1
PUBLIC ATTITUDES TOWARD THE U.S. HEALTH CARE SYSTEM, 1982–1994
(percent)

QUESTION: Which of the following statements comes closest to expressing your overall view of the country's health care system— on the whole, the health care system works pretty well and only minor changes are necessary to make it work better; there are some good things in our health care system, but fundamental changes are needed to make it better; our health care system has so much wrong with it that we need to completely rebuild it?

	Minor Changes Needed	Fundamental Changes	Completely Rebuild
1982	19	47	28
1983	21	50	25
1984	26	49	21
1987	29	47	19
1988	10	60	29
1990	16	59	24
1991	6	50	42
1993	13	49	35
1994	14	54	31

SOURCE: Surveys by Louis Harris and Associates, latest that of April 4–7, 1994.

An ingenious way of asking about the system in laymen's language was provided by ABC News/*Washington Post* pollsters in February and June 1994: "If the health care system were a car, would you say it needs a major overhaul or a good tuneup?" In February, 51 percent said the system needed a major overhaul; 58 percent gave that response in June. In both iterations of the question, about four in ten said a good tuneup would do (see table 2). Americans clearly recognized that our system has many strengths, but substantial numbers said that it also needs work. This evaluation applies to many other areas of American life besides health care. When asked by the Roper Organization in 1993 whether major, minor, or no real changes were needed in a number of American institutions and systems, solid majorities of Americans said major changes were needed in our health care (75 percent), welfare (73 percent), prison (66 percent), tax (64 percent), public education (62 percent), and legal (58 percent) systems. In a poll con-

TABLE 2
PUBLIC EVALUATIONS OF THE U.S. HEALTH CARE SYSTEM, JUNE 1994
(percent)

QUESTION: If the health care system were a car, would you say it needs:

What the System Needs	Feb. 1994	June 1994
A major overhaul	51	58
Good tuneup	44	38
Nothing/leave it alone (vol.)	2	1
Junk it/get a new car/replace it (vol.)	2	2

NOTE: vol. = volunteered response.
SOURCE: Survey by ABC News/*Washington Post*, latest that of June 23–26, 1994.

ducted by the Gallup Organization for CNN and *USA Today* in January 1994, 90 percent of Americans said there was a welfare crisis in the country; 84 percent felt that way about health care. Over and over again, surveys reveal broad concern about the way many central institutions and programs in our country are performing. These answers are admonitions to leaders in the public and private sectors to perform better.

As the debate on health care wound down in the summer and early fall of 1994, most polls showed that Americans wanted to make minor and not major changes in the system. This sentiment reflected unease about what might pass, but it also underscored appreciation of a system with strengths that might be compromised by change. In a September 6–7, 1994, Gallup poll for CNN and *USA Today*, only 20 percent wanted to pass a major reform bill this year, while a plurality (43 percent) wanted to pass minor reforms but to continue working toward major reforms. Seven percent wanted minor reforms and no action next year, and 27 percent wanted the system left as it is.

NBC News/*Wall Street Journal* poll findings in May, June, and July 1994 affirm the response. In each iteration of the question, about six in ten Americans said Congress should debate the issue of health care reform and pass a bill next year. A survey fielded in late August by Yankelovich Partners for *Time* and CNN found 47 percent of Americans saying that the government should "make small changes in our health care system this year and stop there," while 28 percent wanted to wait until next year and try again to make

5

major reform. Two in ten said the government should "stop trying to make reforms and leave the health system as it is." On election day, in the national exit poll conducted by Voter New Service (VNS) for the four networks and AP, 58 percent of voters said that Congress's decision to put off health care was "good because more time is needed for discussion." Thirty-nine percent said this was "bad because the country needs reform now."

Another way of looking at the public's desire for sweeping or incremental reform was provided by the University of Cincinnati's Institute for Policy Research in its survey for the Medical Center conducted in January 1994. In that survey, 72 percent of Americans agreed with this statement: "As far as I am personally concerned, the *only thing* we absolutely must change in the U.S. health care system is the possibility of individuals and families being driven into bankruptcy or poverty by enormous medical bills." Only 17 percent disagreed.

Personal Satisfaction. People's largely positive assessment of their own care contributed to the public's verdict on the 1993–1994 reform effort. When Yankelovich Partners asked Americans in September 1993 how satisfied they were with "the health services which are available to [them] now," the pollsters found 80 percent reporting satisfaction; 16 percent dissented. The Roper Organization has data extending over twenty years on questions relating to both the quality and the availability of care that individuals receive. In 1973, for example, 83 percent of Americans reported that they were very or fairly well satisfied with the quality of the medical care they received. Two decades later, the percentage was 73 percent. Impressions on "availability of medical care when you need it" were similarly high and even more stable. In 1973, three-quarters reported being satisfied with availability; in 1993, the percentage was 74 percent (see table 3). Virtually every survey that has included questions about the quality and availability of health care finds substantial satisfaction.

One area stands out in which the public is clearly unhappy, and it should not surprise us. When asked by the Roper Organization in 1973 whether the cost of medical care they receive is reasonable or unreasonable, 42 percent indicated that the cost was reasonable, but 55 percent disagreed. In 1993, the numbers did not look much different: 40 percent reasonable, 56 percent unreasonable (see table 3). In a survey taken November 8–9, 1994, by the bipartisan polling team of Public Opinion Strategies and Hamilton & Staff, 31 percent of those who indicated that they voted said that health care costs that are too high constitute the "most important health care problem facing the country." This reason was cited by more respondents than any other

TABLE 3
PUBLIC RATINGS OF SATISFACTION WITH ITS MEDICAL CARE, 1973 AND 1993
(percent)

QUESTION: Thinking about all your medical needs, not just the doctor, generally speaking, how satisfied would you say you are with the quality of the medical care you get—very satisfied, fairly well satisfied, not too satisfied, or not at all satisfied?

QUESTION: And how satisfied are you with the availability of medical care when you need it...?

QUESTION: How do you feel about the cost of the medical care you receive—do you feel the cost is very reasonable, fairly reasonable, somewhat unreasonable, or very unreasonable?

Degree of Satisfaction	1973	1993
Satisfied with the quality of medical care you get	83	73
Not satisfied	16	25
Satisfied with the availability of medical care when you need it	75	74
Not satisfied	21	23
Feel the cost of the medical care you receive is unreasonable	55	56
Reasonable	42	40

SOURCE: Surveys by the Roper Organization (Roper Reports 93–9), latest that of September 11–18, 1993.

in the survey. Interestingly, one of the factors that may influence support for universal coverage is concern about cost. Martilla & Kiley, Inc., and the Harvard University School of Public Health's Program on Public Opinion and Health Care asked Americans (for the Robert Wood Johnson Foundation) in March 1993 what arguments would make them feel more or less inclined to support health care reform that would "provide care for all Americans." The highest response category of seven in reflecting people's inclination to support reform was the one that stated, "If all Americans had access to health care, they'd be more likely to get preventive treatment before their health problems get serious and that would keep health care costs lower in the long run." So cost is a significant issue for Americans.

TABLE 4

PUBLIC ESTIMATION OF ABILITY TO HANDLE COSTS OF MAJOR ILLNESS,
1991 AND 1993
(percent)

QUESTION: If a major illness were to occur in your family, could you handle the costs easily, with great difficulty, or probably not at all?

Degree of Difficulty	1991	1993
If a major illness were to occur in family, could handle costs easily	36	34
With difficulty	41	45
Not at all	19	20

SOURCE: Surveys by Yankelovich Partners for *Time* and CNN, latest that of September 23, 1993.

The level of concern about cost has to be put into perspective, however. Most Americans feel pretty confident that they can meet ordinary health care expenses. In 1991, Roper asked Americans this question: "Different people worry about different things when it comes to having enough money to pay for things. Here is a list of some of them. Would you read down that list and tell me for each one whether it is at the present time a major concern of yours, a minor concern, or not a concern?" Having enough money to live on in retirement was seen as a major concern by 50 percent of the population, while far fewer, 37 percent, felt that way about being able to pay for major household repairs. Where did paying for ordinary medical bills rank in this list? Thirty-eight percent said this was a major concern, but 58 percent said it was "minor" or "not a concern." In a question asked in the Martilla & Kiley/Harvard survey described above, Americans were asked how much of a problem it was for them to pay their monthly health insurance premium. Seventy-one percent said it was not a problem or much of a problem. Only 9 percent said it was a serious problem.

Catastrophic expenses are quite different, and poll after poll reveals substantial concern about being able to cover those costs for oneself or one's family. Yankelovich Partners asked Americans in 1991 and twice in 1993 whether they could handle the costs of a major illness in the family easily, with difficulty, or not at all. The responses have hardly varied, as table 4 shows. About a third say they could meet those expenses easily, and two in ten say they could not meet them. Slightly more than 40 percent say they could meet them with difficulty. In the January 1994 survey conducted by the University of Cincinnati for its Medical Center, 77 percent agreed (61 percent of them strongly) that one of their biggest fears about health care is that they or someone in their family "will be financially ruined by large medical bills."

Economic Insecurity. Concern about the cost of health care generally, the ability to manage catastrophic expenses, and economic prospects are a potent admixture, and together they fuel economic insecurity. Richard Curtin, who directs the University of Michigan's consumer confidence survey (which has been tapping the consumer's pulse since 1954), argues that the psychology of prosperity that sustained Americans through the normal ups and downs of the business cycle has eroded substantially. This is evident from polling data today. As this is being written in early November 1994, the country is in the third year of an economic recovery. Yet 54 percent of Americans told Yankelovich Partners (for *Time* and CNN) in early October that the recession had not ended where they live.

Even though Americans see the economy as a whole improving, there is still much underlying anxiety about individual prospects. Thus, concerns about how health care reform would affect their jobs and their wallets loomed large for Americans during this debate. In another question from the January 1994 University of Cincinnati poll, 69 percent disagreed (42 percent of them strongly) that "employers should be required to pay health insurance premiums for all their employees, even if some employees need to be laid off because of the increased costs of business." Only 28 percent agreed employers should be required to pay the premiums in these circumstances.

In April, pollsters from CBS News and the *New York Times* asked 484 senior corporate executives, "If the Clinton plan passes, is it likely that your company will add more jobs as a result, reduce jobs as a result, or don't you think the plan will have any effect on the number of jobs in your company?" Only 3 percent said the bill would cause their companies to add jobs, but 44 percent said it would cause their companies to reduce the number of jobs. A plurality, 49 percent, said passage would not have any effect on the number of jobs in their companies. Virtually identical majorities in June (55 percent) and July (58 percent) 1994 told interviewers from NBC News and the *Wall Street Journal* that costs would increase under the plan. The Clinton plan fueled economic anxiety, and it lost favor.

The inexorable impact of demographic change is affecting concerns about health care, too. In response to a question asked in 1991 by CBS News and the *New York Times*, 48 percent of Americans said that in the next four years, it was likely that "a parent, spouse, or another close relative might need long-term care in a nursing home or some place like that." Of this group, a majority said that they were extremely or very concerned about being able to pay for such care. In March 1993, when Martilla & Kiley/Harvard provided a list of benefits not included in many current plans and asked Americans if they would be willing to pay higher insurance premiums to add each benefit to their own coverage, nursing home care was mentioned more often than any other benefit—including such desirable ones as major medical–catastrophic and prescription drug coverage, to name only two others on the list that some people already had.

Also contributing to insecurity is the fact that many Americans say their health care benefits have been cut back by their employers in the past year. The Roper Organization began asking Americans in 1973 whether they and their families had any type of health care plan or hospital insurance, and the organization has repeated that question six times since. In 1973, 89 percent of Americans said they had coverage; in September 1993, the figure was 82 percent. Total coverage may have declined only slightly, but concerns about cutbacks in current and future coverage appear significant. When Yankelovich Partners asked Americans in September 1993 whether the company they worked for had ever cut or attempted to cut their health benefits, 18 percent of those whose health insurance was provided by an employer answered in the affirmative. But 31 percent of those currently covered said they expected their employer to cut their benefits back in the future.

When asked by CBS News/*New York Times* pollsters in September 1993 and again in March 1994, nearly half the public said they were concerned that someone in their household could be without health insurance in the next five years because of illness or switching jobs. Seventeen percent in the March survey said that someone in their household had been denied coverage because of a preexisting condition. One in three said someone in their household had been without medical coverage at some time in the past twelve months. These numbers bounce around from poll to poll and should not be read literally, but they reveal an anxiety about health care coverage that looms large in what the public perceives as a shaky economic environment.

Surveys began to suggest during the winter and spring of 1994 that the health care issue was losing some of its urgency as a public opinion concern. In 1992, the economy received the lion's share of news coverage, and it generally ranked as the most important issue facing the country. Health care was generally mentioned in a distant second or third position. But as perceptions of the nation's economy's improvement became more widespread, the economy moved from its spot as the most important problem, and another issue, crime, overtook it. Health care moved down the list again. By March 1994, surveyors at Princeton Survey Research Associates (polling for the Times Mirror Center for the People and the Press) reported that even though "personal concern about health care and direct experience with the problems that beset the American health care system rival fear of crime and job problems," the issue was "losing its edge." Times Mirror reported that the public was "backing off key features of reform compared to a year ago."

The Yankelovich surveys for *Time* and CNN presented a similar picture. In September 1993, the economy and unemployment and jobs were cited by 25 percent of Americans as composing the main problem facing the country, and health care was mentioned by 13 percent. Crime was cited by 14 percent. In October 1994, crime was cited by 19 percent, the economy and unemployment and jobs at 15 percent, and health care at just 4 percent. In the five iterations of this question since January 1994, health care consistently ranked below 10 percent as the country's main problem. When asked in a number of different polls what the administration's priorities would be in 1994, Americans ranked crime first, with welfare or health reform second. When people feared losing their jobs, concern about losing health care benefits loomed very large. When immediate concerns about job loss lessened, so did concerns about losing health coverage. This occurred as public doubts about the Clinton health plan were becoming more apparent.

Throughout the 1993–1994 debate over health care reform, Americans indicated to the pollsters that health care would be an important issue to them in casting their votes in November, but that there would be other issues that were important, too. In November 1993, two-thirds told CBS News/*New York Times* pollsters that health care was important but that other issues were important, too. Only 9 percent said it would be the most important issue in determining their vote (see table 5). In a poll taken by Gallup for CNN and *USA Today* in August 1994, 16 percent of Americans said that a candidate's stand on health care would be one of the most important issues they would consider, 54 percent said it would be very important, 24 percent moderately important, and 3 percent not important at all. The figures for the crime bill were 20 percent, 56 percent, 19 percent, and 3 percent. In an October 1994 NBC News/*Wall Street Journal* poll, 33 percent of registered voters said crime would be the most or one of the two most important issues in the election, followed closely by jobs and economic growth at 28 percent; welfare reform, 28 percent; health care, 26 percent; and taxes and government spending, 25 percent. The fact that the issues were closely clustered together in both polls suggested that they are all important to voters.

Another question in the NBC News/*Wall Street Journal* poll asked registered voters which positions would make them "much

TABLE 5

PUBLIC APPRAISAL OF THE IMPORTANCE OF THE HEALTH CARE ISSUE IN
ITS CHOICE OF CONGRESSMEN, NOVEMBER 1993
(percent)

QUESTION: When your representative in the U.S. House of
Representatives runs for reelection next year, how much will your
vote be influenced by his or her position on health care—1, it is the
most important single issue, OR 2, it is important, but so are other
issues, OR 3, it won't influence my vote?

Importance	Percent
Health care is the most important single issue	9
Important, but other issues are too	67
Won't influence	20

SOURCE: Survey by CBS News/*New York Times*, November 11–14, 1993.

more likely to support a candidate"; 49 percent said that support of
the death penalty and "three strikes and you're out" legislation
would make them much more likely to support him or her, 47 percent said a vote to ban assault weapons would make them much
more likely to support the candidate, while far fewer Americans, 31
percent, said working to pass a health care reform bill would make
them much more likely to support the candidate. The issue would
be important, but so would other issues.

General Concerns

Knowing how the public assessed its health care coverage was
essential to understanding how the health care debate developed,
but so too was understanding the predispositions Americans
brought to their thinking about health care. These fundamental predispositions provide the context in which any health care reform
plans in the future will be evaluated by the public.

The Promise of Government. Solid majorities have long told the
pollsters that the nation is spending "too little" on improving and
protecting the nation's health. This is an important value to our
polity, and we expect the government to play a major role in
achieving it. Because health expenses are often a result of things
beyond an individual's control, however, Americans are disposed
toward more government involvement in this area than in areas

TABLE 6

PUBLIC ATTITUDE TOWARD GOVERNMENTAL RESPONSIBILITY FOR
PROVIDING HEALTH CARE, 1938 AND 1991

(percent)

QUESTION: Do you think the government should be responsible for
providing medical care for people who are unable to pay for it?

Government Responsibility	1938	1991
Government should be responsible for providing medical care for people who are unable to pay for it	81	80

SOURCE: Surveys by the Gallup Organization, latest that of June 27–30, 1991.

where individual responsibility is considered greater.

Two questions from the National Opinion Research Center (NORC) about the proper role of government in our society illustrate the point. NORC frames one question this way: "Some people think that the government in Washington should do everything possible to improve the standard of living of all poor Americans—they are at point 1 on this card"; it continues, "Other people think it is not the government's responsibility, and that each person should take care of himself—they are at point 5." NORC asks Americans where they would place themselves on the scale. In terms of improving the living standards of all poor Americans, most people in 1993 placed themselves at point 3, in the middle. The opinions of those who favored a stronger government role and those who said this is not government's responsibility were evenly split.

This split reflects the emphasis Americans give to both individual responsibility and governmental involvement. But when asked about the federal government's responsibility "to see to it that people have help in paying for doctors and hospital care" versus people's taking care of these things themselves, the public was lopsidedly (51 percent) in favor of governmental involvement. A significant number did come down in the middle (32 percent), though, agreeing with both formulations of the issue. Only 16 percent said this was something people should take care of themselves. This question does not explicitly mention people who cannot take care of themselves, and support for a governmental role is still significant.

Health care problems are frequently seen as lying beyond an individual's control, and a compassionate public wants government to step in. This explains the rock-solid responses to a question Gallup first posed in 1938 and repeated again in 1991. In 1938, when Gallup first asked Americans whether government should be responsible for providing medical care for people who are unable to pay for it, 81 percent of Americans agreed. Fifty-three years later, a virtually identical 80 percent of Americans gave the same response (see table 6). Americans expect government involvement in the provision of health care, and they are strongly committed to providing health care for those who cannot provide it for themselves. Still, recognition of individual responsibility will always be a factor in a polity as committed to that core idea as America is. In a survey conducted by Princeton Survey Research Associates for Times Mirror in late March 1994, 35 percent of those surveyed said government should be "most responsible for making sure Americans are covered by health insurance," 31 percent said individuals and their families should be responsible, and 21 percent said the responsibility should be the employers'. In a reflection of persisting partisan differences, Republicans said individuals and their families were most responsible, and Democrats believed government was. Independents split evenly.

Does insistence on universal coverage follow from a conviction about a strong governmental role in the area? And how should the public's support for universal coverage be understood, given the role the public wants government to play in this area? The polls were illuminating here. When asked by Gallup in January 1994 whether they would support a health reform package that guarantees every American private health insurance that can never be taken away, 79 percent agreed, and only 16 percent opposed the idea (see table 7). The importance Americans place on the goal can be seen in answers to the next question in the Gallup battery (also shown in the table): "Suppose Congress passes a bill that would improve the country's health care system, but would not guarantee coverage for every American. Do you think President Clinton should veto the bill and send it back to Congress, or should he sign it?" Seventy-three percent said he should veto it, and only 22 percent said he should sign it. Proceeding along, Americans indicated in the next question that they would still support the idea if taxes were going to go up. These three questions reveal deep support for the goal. But other values or concerns temper support for universal coverage. When asked in the same battery of questions whether they would still favor guaranteed coverage "if [they] thought that the availability of health services would be limited," respondents turned decisively against the idea of guaranteed coverage, with 69 percent opposing it and only 26 percent favoring it (see table 7).

A question asked by Yankelovich Partners for *Time* and CNN

TABLE 7

PUBLIC RESPONSES TO QUESTIONS ABOUT GUARANTEED COVERAGE, 1994
(percent)

Question	Percent		

QUESTION: Would you *support* or *oppose* a health care reform package that guarantees every American private health insurance that can never be taken away?

	Aug.	*June*	*Jan.*
Support	69	77	79
Oppose	24	17	16

QUESTION: Suppose Congress passes a bill which would *improve* the country's health care system, but would *not* guarantee *coverage* for every American. Do you think President Clinton should *veto* the bill and send it back to Congress, or should he *sign* it?

Veto bill	NA	70	73
Sign it		20	22

QUESTION: If guaranteed coverage for every American is adopted, some people say it could cause individual Americans' taxes to go up. Would you still favor guaranteed coverage if you thought that individual Americans' taxes would go up, or not?

Yes, favor	NA	NA	72
No, oppose			25

QUESTION: Suppose the effect of guaranteed coverage was to limit the availability of health services. Would you still favor guaranteed coverage if you thought that the availability of health services would be limited, or not?

Yes, favor	NA	NA	26
No, oppose			69

NOTE: NA = Not asked.
SOURCE: Survey by the Gallup Organization for *USA Today* and CNN, latest that of August 1994.

TABLE 8

PUBLIC ATTITUDES TOWARD RAISING TAXES TO PROVIDE
HEALTH INSURANCE FOR ALL AMERICANS, 1994
(percent)

QUESTION: Would you prefer a health reform plan that raises taxes in order to provide health insurance to all Americans, or a plan that does not provide health insurance to all Americans but keeps taxes at current levels?

Preferred Plan	Feb.	June
Raises taxes; health care for all	46	43
Keeps taxes at current level; no health care for all	42	44

SOURCE: Surveys by Yankelovich Partners for *Time* and CNN, latest that of June 1994.

in February 1994 and again in June shows how changes in wording and emphasis can influence public thinking about the goal of universal coverage. This is a question about the tax burden that universal coverage could impose. The question divided Americans in both iterations, and in June, 43 percent of Americans said they would prefer a health plan that raises taxes to provide health insurance for all Americans, while 44 percent said they would prefer a plan that does not provide health insurance to all but keeps taxes at current levels (see table 8). A generous public feels strapped in an era of economic anxiety.

Some polls, such as the Gallup one cited above, suggested strong support for the president's commitment to veto legislation that did not include universal coverage, while others indicated that this issue should not hold up progress on reform. A question asked by NBC News and the *Wall Street Journal* in March 1994, for example, may have captured that sentiment. The surveyors found that 47 percent of Americans said the president should refuse to sign a health care bill that would not provide universal coverage for all Americans, but a significant 43 percent said he should sign it (see table 9).

Another way of looking at the importance of universal coverage is provided by examining how the public ranks this goal in comparison with other concerns. The bipartisan polling team of Mellman/Lazarus/Lake and the Tarrance Group, polling for *U.S. News & World Report*, asked Americans in January 1994: "As a goal, how important to you is it that every American have health care

TABLE 9

PUBLIC ATTITUDE TOWARD A HEALTH CARE REFORM BILL NOT
GUARANTEEING UNIVERSAL COVERAGE, MARCH 1994

(percent)

QUESTION: Should President Clinton refuse to sign a health care
reform bill that would not provide universal health coverage for all
Americans?

Should Clinton Refuse to Sign?	Percent
Yes	47
No	43

SOURCE: Survey by NBC News/*Wall Street Journal*, March 4–8, 1994.

coverage?" Twenty percent said it was one of their top goals, 44
percent said a very important goal, 22 percent said somewhat
important. Only 6 percent said it was not at all important (see table
10). In the Martilla & Kiley/Harvard poll done in March 1993, 83
percent of Americans said that making sure that those who now
have coverage do not lose it when they change jobs, get laid off, or
retire was a very important goal; in comparison, 72 percent said
that providing coverage for those who are now uninsured was a
very important goal for them.

Other questions reveal more about Americans' priorities.
Yankelovich Partners polling for *Time* and CNN in February 1994,
asked which was the bigger problem—that health care coverage is
not available to everyone, or that the costs of health care coverage
are too high. A decisive 67 percent said the bigger problem was cost.
Far fewer, 27 percent, said the bigger problem was coverage not
being available (see table 11). Martilla & Kiley/Harvard polling in
March 1993 reinforces the point. In this poll, 54 percent said the
biggest problem with our health care system is that "costs are too
high," 23 percent said that "too many Americans have no health
insurance at all," and 15 percent said that it is "when people lose
their jobs, they usually lose their health insurance." In a September
1994 CBS News/*New York Times* poll, 76 percent of Americans said
it was very important that every American receive health insurance
coverage, but 81 percent said it was very important that any health
care plan provide insurance that Americans cannot lose. In another
question posing a trade-off, 45 percent of Americans told ABC
News/*Washington Post* pollsters that "guaranteeing health insurance
for all Americans whether they can pay for it or not" was more

TABLE 10
PUBLIC EVALUATION OF IMPORTANCE OF UNIVERSAL COVERAGE,
JANUARY 1994
(percent)

QUESTION: As a goal, how important to you is it that every American have health coverage?

Universal Coverage	Percent
One of my top goals	20
Very important	44
Somewhat important	22
Not very important	6
Not at all important	6

SOURCE: Survey by Mellman/Lazarus/Lake and the Tarrance Group for *U.S. News & World Report,* January 17–18, 1994.

important to them, while 49 percent said "holding down the cost of health care for working people" was more important. Writing in the spring 1994 issue of *Health Affairs,* Robert Blendon and others involved in the Harvard project describe universal coverage as a "core" value, but they also say it "is not enough to generate popular support for a national health care program." The subsequent debate proved them correct. Universal coverage is a goal and has been for a long time, but it is tempered by other considerations, most notably concern about costs and limitations on care.

Responses to questions that ask how much more Americans would be willing to pay in federal income taxes to ensure that all would be covered fluctuate considerably, and they should not be read literally. These questions ask for precision that is unrealistic in surveys, and they fail to take into account Americans' cumulative tax burden. Even though the Clinton administration argued that most Americans' taxes did not go up when they filled out their returns this year, polls consistently show that Americans believe their taxes went up. A poll conducted by Princeton Survey Research Associates for *Newsweek* in October 1994, for example, found that a majority of Americans said taxes had gone up on the middle class. Americans usually think about their tax burden in total and do not separate federal, state, local, property, sales, and other taxes into discrete categories.

But the relevant point here is that the public's commitment to universal coverage is not open-ended. Most Americans say they

TABLE 11
PUBLIC RANKING OF THE PROBLEMS OF AVAILABILITY OF
COVERAGE AND HIGH COSTS, FEBRUARY 1994
(percent)

QUESTION: Which do you think is a bigger problem—that health care coverage is not available to everyone, or that the costs of health care are too high?

Bigger Problem	Percent
Coverage not available to everyone	27
Costs too high	67

SOURCE: Survey by Yankelovich Partners for *Time* and CNN, February 10, 1994.

would be willing to pay more for the uninsured to receive coverage, but there are limits. In one poll, of those who said they would be willing to pay more for universal coverage (65 percent of those surveyed), 95 percent said they would pay $10 more a month to accomplish the goal, 61 percent said $30 more a month, and 39 percent would pay $50 more a month (Martilla & Kiley/Harvard).

Researchers at the University of Cincinnati found in January 1994 that nearly half of all Americans (48 percent) were willing to pay higher federal and state taxes to guarantee that "all U.S. citizens have health insurance coverage," but 40 percent said they were not willing. When the university researchers asked a follow-up question about how much more people would be willing to pay each year in taxes for universal coverage, 42 percent indicated that they would not be willing to pay anything more each year, 7 percent said less than $100 a year, 13 percent between $100 and $299 a year, and 11 percent $300 a year or more. Twenty-eight percent said they did not know. While polls vary on where Americans draw the line in terms of willingness to pay more in taxes, limits exist.

The Problem of Government. Counterbalancing the substantial role most Americans see for government in health care provision is the considerable skepticism they have about government's abilities to perform well in the area. Americans are profoundly ambivalent about government, particularly the federal government. On the one hand, they think that government should do many things in such a rich and powerful country as our own. On the other, they see government as problem causing. The weight of polling evidence today is clearly on the latter view of government. Americans do not viscerally oppose government involvement in their lives, but they viscerally oppose the incompetence government projects today.

Many Clinton supporters argue that Bill Clinton's election was a decisive endorsement of a more assertive role for government in our society. It may have been a rejection of the supine role for government that George Bush seemed to project, but it was not an endorsement for its antithesis. When voters were asked by the exit pollsters on election day 1992 whether they wanted a bigger government with more services and higher taxes or a smaller government with fewer services and lower taxes, only Bill Clinton's supporters opted for a bigger government with more services and higher taxes. Supporters of George Bush and Ross Perot decisively "voted" for smaller government. The exit pollsters did not repeat this question in 1994, but a similar one makes the same point. In the national exit poll conducted by Voter News Service (the exit poll consortium of the four networks and AP), a decisive 56 precent said government is doing too many things better left to business and individuals; 41 percent said government should do more to solve national problems. The election results suggested a desire for smaller government. In his postelection news conference, even President Clinton agreed with this assessment: "They're [the American people] still not sure that we understand what they expect the role of government to be. I think they want a smaller government that gives them better value for their dollar, that reflects both their interests and their values, that is not a burden to them but that empowers them."

The dissatisfaction with government performance today permeates and influences public concerns about new federal involvement in health care. In a session with reporters mentioned in the *Wall Street Journal* after the demise of the Clinton plan, Health and Human Services Secretary Donna Shalala suggested the administration would scale back its health care reform approach in 1995. According to the *Journal's* brief, one-page account, Shalala said that Americans feared that the administration would have instituted a government-run system and that it hoped to avoid what she called "that handicap" in the future.

The polls showed that this fear resonated with Americans almost immediately in the debate. Using a unique, in-depth survey approach, the Public Agenda Foundation questioned 564 people in thirteen cities in November 1993 and then, after an hour-long educational effort, questioned them again. Skepticism about governmental performance was overwhelming. One man from Denver said, "Any time the government is in it, it is going to get worse." A Virginia woman thought ahead: "If you let the government take control away from you, it's hard to get it back." A Boston man com-

TABLE 12
PUBLIC ESTIMATION OF GOVERNMENT INVOLVEMENT CREATED BY
CLINTON PLAN, SEPTEMBER 1993–MARCH 1994
(percent)

QUESTION: Do you think Clinton's plan creates too much government involvement in the nation's health care system, not enough government involvement, or about the right amount?

	Too Much Involvement	Not Enough	About the Right Amount
Sept. 1993	38	18	37
Oct. 1993	40	18	37
Nov. 1993	46	15	33
Jan. 1994	40	12	39
Feb. 1994	42	16	38
Mar. 1994	47	14	34

SOURCE: Surveys by ABC News/*Washington Post*, latest that of March 25–27, 1994.

mented: "I just hate the idea of giving government something else to work on."

A plurality of Americans consistently told the pollsters that the Clinton plan "create[d] too much government involvement in the nation's health care system" (see table 12). In the last asking of that question in the March 1994 ABC News/*Washington Post* poll, 47 percent said too much, 14 percent said not enough, and 34 percent said about the right amount. When asked by these pollsters in February 1994 about big, small, or nonexistent concerns they had about the Clinton health care plan, 62 percent acknowledged as a big concern that the plan would "create another large and inefficient government bureaucracy." Only 14 percent said that was not a concern (see table 13). When asked in September 1994 by CBS News/*New York Times* interviewers to select among five major or minor reasons (another category was "not a reason") why health care reform did not pass, 56 percent cited as a major reason that the plan had too much government involvement, 56 percent said special interests and lobbyists did not want health care passed, 51 percent that the Republicans blocked action, 50 percent that the Democrats were split, and 46 percent that the president's plan was too complicated. The closeness of these responses indicates a public verdict of multiple reasons, but it is still significant that too much

21

TABLE 13

PUBLIC CONCERN OVER GOVERNMENT BUREAUCRACY BY CLINTON PLAN,
FEBRUARY 1994

(percent)

QUESTION: Now I'm going to mention things that might concern some people but not others about the Clinton health care plan. And for each, please tell me if it's a big concern, a small concern, or not at all a concern of yours. Here's the first: The plan would create another large and inefficient government bureaucracy.

Degree of Concern	Percent
Big concern	62
Small concern	23
Not a concern	14

SOURCE: Survey by ABC News/*Washington Post*, February 24–27, 1994.

government involvement tied for first place.

In a question asked in 1992 and not repeated since then, Mellman/Lazarus and Public Opinion Strategies asked Americans about what the results might be of instituting a government-run national health insurance program. Significant numbers did not have opinions, but 53 percent said there would be less freedom of choice, only 12 percent said more freedom; 47 percent said there would be more delays, 13 percent said fewer; 37 percent said the quality of health care would be lower, 13 percent said higher; 30 percent said that there would be less access to the health care that people need, 16 percent said more; 36 percent said there would be less flexibility, 19 percent said more; 42 percent said health care would be more costly, while 25 percent said it would be less costly. The only "positive" aspect seen in a government-run plan, and it was not overwhelming, was that general fairness would be improved. Forty-three percent of Americans said it would be better, but nearly a quarter, 23 percent, said that fairness would be worse too (see table 14). The Public Agenda researchers concluded from their study that the public was "extremely dubious" about the role of government in reforming health care, particularly in the area of holding down costs.

Those who see the public's view of government's role more robustly point to polls showing considerable skepticism about other big players in the health care field—the American Medical Association and the health insurance industry, to name just two.

TABLE 14
PUBLIC ATTITUDES TOWARD VARIOUS FEATURES OF A NATIONAL HEALTH
INSURANCE PROGRAM, JANUARY 1992
(percent)

QUESTION: If a government-run national health insurance program were in place, do you think...would be...?

Features	Percent
Overall fairness would be...	
better	43
worse	23
Health care would be...	
less costly	25
more costly	42
Degree of flexibility would be...	
greater	19
less	36
To medical care you need, there would be...	
more access	16
less access	30
Quality would be...	
higher	13
lower	37
Delays would be...	
fewer	13
more	47
Freedom of choice would be...	
more	12
less	53

SOURCE: Survey by Mellman/Lazarus and Public Opinion Strategies for the Health Insurance Association of America, January 4–5, 1992.

Americans are clearly skeptical about big, powerful institutions, so it is not surprising to find this sentiment in the polls. In the February, July, and August 1994 ABC News/*Washington Post* polls, for example, slightly more than 60 percent of Americans said the health insurance industry was hurting efforts to improve the nation's health care system. Fifty-two, 50, and 48 percent, respectively, felt that way about the American Medical Association. And, in a September 1994 poll taken by CBS News and the *New York Times*, a solid majority (56 percent) gave as a reason for the defeat of the Clinton plan the presence of special interests and lobbyists who did not want health care reform.

Still, business is generally seen as far more able than government. In a Roper Organization poll conducted in January 1988 and not updated since then, 74 percent of Americans said that business was run more efficiently, while only 9 percent felt that way about federal agencies. When asked by the National Opinion Research Center about their confidence in major companies, 21 percent indicated in 1993 that they had "a great deal" of confidence; only 7 percent felt that way about Congress. Twelve percent had "hardly any" confidence in major companies, but 41 percent had hardly any confidence in Congress. Paradoxically, because business outperforms government in the public's mind, the public may be disposed to place more responsibility on employers in the provision of health care.

The Importance of Choice. One of the most powerful currents in our democracy is the importance of individual choice. The sentiment comes up in polling questions about education, the decision to have an abortion, whether or not to allow individuals to smoke, and even whether to allow individuals to end their own lives. We see the same powerful sentiment in the importance Americans place on being able to choose their own doctors. In the Public Agenda study, researchers found that "the importance people attach to a personal relationship with a physician came up repeatedly." This was a far higher goal than access to the most up-to-date hospitals, research, and experimental procedures. Public Agenda concluded that "to the degree that patients sense that doctors don't have enough time for them or that they are continually running cost calculations in their heads, the reformed health care system may be interpreted as violating one of the most central of the American public's values."

Reinforcing this opinion are the answers to a question posed by ABC News/*Washington Post* pollsters in February 1994 and several times before. Asked whether they would choose an expensive plan that allows them to choose their own doctors or an inexpensive program that does not allow them to choose their own doctors, the public opted decisively for choosing their own doctors, even if that would be expensive (see table 15). ABC News/*Washington Post* polling in April and September of 1993 and February and June of

TABLE 15

PUBLIC APPRAISAL OF VALUE OF FREEDOM TO CHOOSE DOCTORS, 1991–1994
(percent)

QUESTION: Which of these would you choose: (read items)

Choice vs. Cost	July 1991	Sept. 1993	Feb. 1994
An inexpensive health care program that does *not* allow you to choose your own doctor	25	32	26
An expensive health care program that allows you to choose your own doctor	69	58	62

SOURCE: Surveys by ABC News/*Washington Post*, latest that of February 24–27, 1994.

1994 puts the issue of choice in another light. In each iteration of this question, 60 percent of Americans said they would favor a program in which people paid more money to choose their own doctor and less money if they went to an assigned doctor. In both October 1993 and August 1994, strong pluralities of Americans (42 and 44 percent, respectively) told Gallup pollsters (in the field for CNN and *USA Today*) that if health care reform passed, they would expect to have fewer choices. Thirty-nine percent in October and 34 percent in August said their choices would be about the same, while only one in five felt in both polls that they would have more choices.

In an effort to expose Americans to methods of saving money used by countries that spend less on health care, the Martilla & Kiley/Harvard team found that 70 percent of Americans rejected a proposal under which "individuals would have a limited choice of doctors and hospitals they could use," even if it would save them money. Only 28 percent endorsed the idea. In the late March 1994 PSRA/Times Mirror survey, 68 percent said they would not be willing to accept more restrictions on their choice of doctors and hospitals in a new health care system; 29 percent said they would be willing to accept this. University of Cincinnati pollsters asked Americans about this issue in a slightly different way in January 1994. They asked whether Americans would accept no limitations, some limitations, or substantial limitations on their primary care doctors, specialists, or hospitals. Twenty-two percent said they would accept no limitations on their primary care doctors, 60 percent some limitations, and 17 percent substantial limitations. The percentages for specialists were 28, 57, and 15, and for hospitals they were 28, 57, and 13 percent.

In March 1994 polling for the *New York Times*, 56 percent of Americans said they could currently choose any doctor at all, 33 percent said they could "choose from a list," and 5 percent said they had no choice at all. It may seem irrelevant to talk about freedom to choose one's own doctor when it appears that this is no longer the reality for many Americans. But the worry appears to come when the government is seen to be further restricting individual choice in this area and others.

The Clinton Plan

Within hours of President Clinton's September speech on health care reform, survey organizations were in the field trying to capture the public's reaction. News organizations reported strong support for the Clinton plan. In fact, no such support existed. Americans' "support" was a response to a very strong speech on a subject of great concern. By equating reactions to a speech with support for the plan, the administration found itself in the unenviable position of having to respond to questions about why support declined. Throughout the debate, Americans knew very little about the Clinton plan. Their answers to questions asked about it (and about competing plans) reflected broad general concerns about the direction any reform effort might have taken.

Many debates in Washington—such as on the reauthorization of Superfund or on having numeric quotas for Japanese products —have been relegated to the domain of experts. While Americans arguably have a more immediate stake in the direction health care reform might take, they were not well informed about specific proposals. In April 1994, seven months after the president's plan was introduced, 73 percent of Americans told CBS News/*New York Times* interviewers that it was "too early" to have a good understanding of what the Clinton health care plan meant, while 25 percent said they already had a good understanding. Only 30 percent of business executives, surveyed by CBS News in April, said that they had a good understanding of what the plan would mean for their business. Sixty percent did not. Polling since the fall of 1993 consistently revealed that a significant number of Americans did not know much about the Clinton proposal (see table 16).

Given the extent to which a president dominates news coverage, it was not surprising that public awareness of competing Republican and Democratic plans was exceedingly low. When asked in December 1993 whether there was a specific Republican plan for health care, 63 percent of Americans told Times Mirror

TABLE 16
PUBLIC ESTIMATION OF ITS UNDERSTANDING OF
CLINTON HEALTH CARE PLAN, SEPTEMBER 1993–APRIL 1994
(percent)

QUESTION: As of now, do you think you have a good understanding of what the Clinton health care plan will mean, or is it too early to know that yet?

	Good Understanding of the Clinton Plan	Too Early to Know
Sept. 1993	13	84
Oct. 6–7	23	75
Oct. 18–19	18	79
Nov.	21	77
Feb. 1994	27	70
April	25	73

QUESTION: How much do you feel you know about Clinton's health care plan—a lot, a little, or do you feel that you know almost nothing about it?

	Know a Lot about the Clinton Plan	A Little	Almost Nothing
Oct. 1993	17	53	30
Feb. 1994	24	62	14

SOURCE: For first question, surveys by the CBS News/*New York Times*, latest that of April 21–23, 1994; for second question, surveys by ABC News/*Washington Post*, latest that of February 24–27, 1994.

interviewers that they did not know of one, 20 percent said there was a proposal, and 17 percent said there was not.

When the president's plan was outlined in September, a number of underlying concerns about reform were brought to the surface. Americans were concerned about the total cost of a new plan and the costs for them, as the data in table 17 show. Given that this issue had stood out in survey data for several decades as a major concern about the health care area generally, this concern was not surprising. In August 1994, 48 percent of Americans told Gallup interviewers polling for CNN and *USA Today* that health care costs

TABLE 17

PUBLIC EXPECTATIONS OF HEALTH CARE COSTS UNDER THE
CLINTON PLAN, SEPTEMBER 1993–MARCH 1994
(percent)

QUESTION: From what you have heard, if the Clinton health care plan is adopted, do you think the amount you pay for the health care you and your family receive will increase, decrease, or stay about the same?

	Increase	Decrease	Stay about the Same
Sept. 1993	45	14	33
Oct. 6–7, 1993	51	13	29
Oct. 18–19, 1993	55	9	29
Nov. 1993	53	9	33
Dec. 1993	55	9	30
Feb. 1994	53	9	31
Mar. 1994	57	11	26

SOURCE: Surveys by CBS News/*New York Times*, latest that of March 8–11, 1994.

under health care reform would "continue to rise out of control." Forty-three percent selected the response that they would "start to get under control." This mirrored findings by other pollsters. When people were asked in a *New York Times* question in March 1994 what their biggest worry was about the Clinton plan and allowed to give any response they wished, "cost" was mentioned more often than any other issue. The numbers of Americans saying that their costs would increase under the plan rose from September onward in CBS News/*New York Times* polling, and the last time they were asked the question, in March 1994, 57 percent said their costs would increase, only 11 percent said they would decrease, and 26 percent said they would remain about the same (see table 17). When Gallup interviewers posed a slightly different variation of this question in September and October 1993 and then again in August 1994, a majority each time said that costs would increase.

Nearly three times as many Americans (34 percent) said in August 1994 that the quality of their care would decrease for "you and your family" as that it would increase (13 percent) (see table 18). There was some indication in the survey data that this issue became more important throughout the debate in 1994. In late

TABLE 18
PUBLIC EXPECTATIONS OF HEALTH CARE QUALITY UNDER THE
CLINTON PLAN, SEPTEMBER 1993–AUGUST 1994
(percent)

QUESTION: From what you have heard, if the Clinton health care plan is adopted, do you think the quality of the health care you and your family receive will increase, decrease, or stay about the same?

	Increase	Decrease	Stay about the Same
Sept. 1993	17	23	53
Oct. 6–7, 1993	16	29	50
Oct. 18–19, 1993	16	32	46
Nov. 1993	15	30	51
Dec. 1993	15	29	51
Feb. 1994	12	31	50
Mar. 1994	11	34	51
Aug. 1994*	13	34	49

NOTE: *Question wording varied slightly. In August, question wording was as follows: "From what you have heard, if Congress adopts a health care reform plan this year, do you think the quality of the health care you and your family receive will increase, decrease, or stay about the same?"
SOURCE: Surveys by CBS News/New York Times, latest that of August 16–17, 1994.

February polling done by ABC News and the Washington Post—polling in which general opposition to the plan outweighed general support for the first time since the news organizations began posing the question in September—the surveyors said that the most notable shift in concerns was "the jump in the number of those saying that they feared that the quality of their own medical care would decline." The number saying this was a big concern was 64 percent in October and 80 percent in February.

Another major concern was fairness. The public was divided throughout the fall of 1993 and the winter of 1994, as table 19 shows, about whether the plan was fair "to people like you," but in April, the last time CBS News and the New York Times posed the question, 48 percent said it would not be fair, while 38 percent said it would. In August, Americans told Gallup that the Clinton health care plan would hurt the middle class disproportionately. When asked "who would be hurt the most by health care reform," 19 percent said upper-class Americans, 38 percent the middle class, and

---

TABLE 19
PUBLIC APPRAISAL OF FAIRNESS OF THE CLINTON PLAN,
SEPTEMBER 1993–APRIL 1994
(percent)

QUESTION: Do you think the health care reform plan Bill Clinton is proposing is fair to people like you, or not?

Date of Poll	Fair	Not Fair
Sept. 1993	40	36
Oct. 6–7, 1993	45	37
Oct. 18–19, 1993	40	40
Nov. 1993	42	39
Dec. 1993	42	41
Jan. 1994	42	43
Feb. 1994	38	44
Mar. 1994	44	40
April 1994	38	48

SOURCE: Surveys by the CBS News/*New York Times*, latest that of April 21–23, 1994.

---

14 percent the poor. Political analyst William Schneider, my colleague at AEI, argues that President Clinton lost the health care reform battle when he lost the support of the middle class on the issue. This group feared that they would not be getting anything that benefited them from reform, and they also felt they could lose some of the benefits they already had.

Other concerns affected public perceptions of the Clinton plan. The February ABC News/*Washington Post* poll found more than two-thirds of Americans identifying the following as big concerns: the plan would cost too much; there would be a lot of fraud and abuse; taxes would have to be increased; some kinds of expensive services would not be available to all who would need them; the cost of one's own care would increase; and finally, the choice of doctors and hospitals might be limited. Given these worries, it should not surprise us that majorities told the pollsters that the more they heard about the plan, the less they liked it (see table 20). Another question asked by Gallup in August 1994 for CNN and *USA Today* found that 48 percent of Americans said the fact that "[their] health care will become worse if Congress passes a health care reform bill this year" worried them more than "that [their] health care will become worse if Congress does not pass a bill this year" (32 percent).

TABLE 20
EVOLVING PUBLIC SENTIMENT CONCERNING CLINTON PLAN, NOVEMBER 1993 AND FEBRUARY 1994
(percent)

QUESTION: Which of these comes closest to your own view:

View	November 1993	February 1994
A. The more I hear about Clinton's health care plan, the more I like it.	41	44
B. The more I hear about Clinton's health care plan, the less I like it.	53	51

SOURCE: Surveys by ABC News/*Washington Post*, latest that of February 24–27, 1994.

The public chorus throughout the debate was: make the system better, but do not destroy or compromise the parts of it that are working well. Answers to questions that asked Americans whether they favored or opposed the Clinton plan were indicators of anxiety about reform (see table 21). Americans told their leaders in Congress to go slowly and to make changes in the Clinton plan. In three differently worded questions that provided trend data on how Congress should have reacted to the Clinton plan, majorities or strong pluralities of Americans continually suggested that changes be made in it (see table 22). Given the doubts about the Clinton plan, it should not surprise us that in August 1994 a decisive 68 percent of Americans told the Gallup Organization that Congress should deal with health care reform on a gradual basis over several years.

The data showed support throughout the debate for the fact that the administration was making an effort in the area, and the Democrats are seen in many but not all polls today as the party better able to handle the issue. In ABC News/*Washington Post* polling, 60 percent in late February, 56 percent in July, and 54 percent in August credited the Clinton administration with helping to improve the system. ABC/*Washington Post* pollsters asked Americans on a number of different occasions whether the Clinton plan was better or worse than the present system. In each of five surveys since September 1993, a majority of Americans said the Clinton plan was better than the current system, although the number saying it was worse doubled (from 17 percent in September to 38 percent in March).

TABLE 21
PUBLIC ATTITUDE TOWARD CLINTON/DEMOCRATIC CONGRESSIONAL HEALTH PLANS, SEPTEMBER 1993–AUGUST 1994
(percent)

QUESTION: From everything you have heard or read about the plan so far, do you favor or oppose President Clinton's plan to reform health care?

Date of Poll	Favor Clinton Plan	Oppose It
Sept. 24–26, 1993	59	33
Oct. 28–30, 1993	45	45
Nov. 2–4, 1993	52	40
Nov. 19–21, 1993	52	41
Jan. 15–17, 1994	56	38
Jan. 28–30, 1994	57	38
Feb. 26–28, 1994	46	48
April 16–18, 1994	43	47
May 20–22, 1994	46	49
June 25–28, 1994	43	49
July 15–17, 1994	40	55
Aug. 8–9, 1994[a]	39	46
Aug. 15–16, 1994[a]	39	48

QUESTION: From what you have heard or read, do you favor or oppose President Clinton's health care program?

Date of Poll	Favor Clinton Plan	Oppose It	Need to Know More (volunteered)
Sept. 22, 1993	51	18	17
Oct. 22–26, 1993	47	37	12
Dec. 11–14, 1993	47	32	15
Jan. 15–18, 1994	42	39	12
Mar. 3–8, 1994	37	45	12
April 30–May 3, 1994	36	44	14
June 10–14, 1994	38	46	11
July 23–26, 1994	41	48	7

TABLE 21 (continued)

QUESTION: From what you know of it, do you approve or disapprove of Clinton's health care plan?

Date of Poll	Approve of Clinton Plan	Disapprove
Sept. 19, 1993	43	41
Sept. 22, 1993	56	24
Oct. 10, 1993	51	39
Nov. 14, 1993	46	43
Jan. 23, 1994	48	39
Feb. 8, 1994	51	41
Feb. 27, 1994	44	48
Mar. 27, 1994	42	48
May 15, 1994	44	50
June 26, 1994	42	53

a. Question wording changed to "Next, thinking about health care, do you favor or oppose the health care reform plans proposed by leaders of the Democratic party in Congress?"
SOURCE: For first question, surveys by the Gallup Organization for *USA Today* and CNN; for second question, surveys by NBC News/*Wall Street Journal*; for third question, surveys by ABC News/*Washington Post*.

Given the lack of knowledge about the plan, the responses to this question were probably an endorsement of the effort to fix a system that has some serious problems, not a definitive evaluation of the Clinton plan. It is also not surprising that in *New York Times* polling in March 1994, 86 percent of Americans said there was not another health care plan they had heard of that they thought would be better than the Clinton plan. The administration's plan looked good by default when there was not much information about other plans.

What Direction Reform? In the Pennsylvania Senate election in 1991 that propelled Democrat Harris Wofford into the U.S. Senate, 60 percent of voters in polling there on November 6–7 endorsed a Canadian national health insurance program for the United States, and an identical 60 percent endorsed a system with a choice of private health plans, along with public plans for the poor and elderly (a description of the U.S. system). That significant numbers of Americans could endorse two different systems by wide margins in questions in the same poll should give pause to anyone claiming

TABLE 22

Public Attitudes about How Congress Should React to the Clinton Plan, September 1993–June 1994

(percent)

QUESTION: Do you think Congress should pass the health care plan basically as Bill Clinton has proposed it, pass it, but only after making changes, or reject this plan?

	Pass Plan	Pass with Major Changes	Reject Plan
Sept. 1993	23	54	15
Oct. 1993	23	45	24
Nov. 1993	24	50	20
Jan. 1994	24	55	16
Feb. 1994	20	47	28
Mar. 1994	19	47	26
April 1994	19	51	23

QUESTION: Based on what you currently know about President Clinton's health care reform plan, do you think Congress should pass that bill in its current form, pass it after making minor changes, pass it after making major changes, or reject the plan completely?

	Pass Plan	Pass with Minor Changes	Pass with Major Changes	Reject Plan
Dec. 1993	9	33	22	25
Feb. 1994	4	37	31	19

QUESTION: What do you think Congress should do with Clinton's health care plan: pass it without any changes, pass it with minor changes, pass it, but with major changes, or not pass any of it?

	Pass Plan	Pass with Minor Changes	Pass with Major Changes	Not Pass Any of It
Sept. 19, 1993	7	39	27	16
Sept. 22, 1993	9	48	23	10
Oct. 10, 1993	5	47	26	18
Nov. 14, 1993	6	42	29	17
Jan. 23, 1994	6	41	26	19
Feb. 27, 1994	4	41	32	19
Mar. 27, 1994	5	44	28	20
May 15, 1994	6	38	27	25
June 26, 1994	4	38	31	22

SOURCE: For first question, surveys by the Gallup Organization for *USA Today* and CNN, latest that of April 16–18, 1994; for second question, surveys by Yankelovich Partners for *Time* and CNN, latest that of February 10, 1994; for third question, surveys by ABC News/*Washington Post*, latest that of June 26, 1994.

that opinion about any proposal is firm. Yet that is precisely what happened in the third wave of polling on health care reform.

Surveys provided a wealth of information on how Americans rated their own care and on their worries about reform. The polls illuminated those concerns. But surveys have their limitations. They are most useful in areas where people bring substantial personal knowledge and experience to an issue and where people identify broad and general policy concerns. They could tell us about the reservations Americans had about the Clinton plan based on their perceptions of their current care and their concerns about what new government involvement would mean for them, but they could not tell us whether President Clinton's health care plan was preferable to those of Representatives Cooper or McDermott or Senators Chafee or Gramm, to name only four of the competing proposals. Yet pollsters in the third wave of surveys began to suggest that this kind of certainty existed.

Certainty did not exist, because knowledge was low. In the Public Agenda exercise, nearly three-quarters of Americans thought that the federal government spent more on humanitarian foreign aid than it did on health care for older people. When Americans were asked by Martilla & Kiley/Harvard in March 1993, 60 percent said they had never heard of the term "managed competition," 63 percent had never heard of "play or pay," and 65 percent had never heard of "single payer." Only 23 percent, 17 percent, and 21 percent, respectively, said they had heard those terms and knew what they meant.

The Harvard Program employed Princeton Survey Research Associates (PSRA) in January 1994 to inquire about three alternatives the survey organization described (single-payer, individual mandates, and employer mandates). Fifty-five, 65, and 44 percent, respectively, indicated that they had not heard or read anything about those alternatives. Yet in the very next question, the surveyors asked Americans which of the three plans they would support if they were casting a vote in a national election! The "employer mandate" proposal "won." Forty percent of Americans "voted" for it, 17 percent supported the individual mandate, and 19 percent liked the single-payer option. An employer mandate probably won because it did not appear to have substantial government involvement or because many Americans already get their coverage through their employers and feel more comfortable with this approach than with unknown alternatives. The plan may also have appeared costless to employees.

In the PSRA/Harvard poll, the employer mandate was described this way: "Under this plan, you pay for health insurance indirectly through your employer. All employers are required to offer health insurance to their workers. Your employer pays a fixed amount of your health insurance costs, while you pay the rest. You are given a choice of private health insurance plans. Small business and low-income individuals are offered a subsidy to help them pay their health insurance bills." The phrasing was an attempt to describe how a complicated proposal would work, but it said nothing about possible consequences of enactment. What if the already complicated wording had included something like the following: "Many experts believe that the wages of some workers will have to go down to pay for the employer mandate." Would the idea of an employer mandate have generated as much support? It is impossible to know, of course, but the exercise shows how problematic this kind of polling can be.

In February, PSRA/Harvard repeated this exercise. In the new poll, they found that 36 percent of Americans had not heard or read about an employer mandate plan, while 63 percent had. (This question cannot be directly compared with the January PSRA question because the wording changed slightly.) In the question that followed this one, however, only 27 percent associated the employer mandate with President Clinton. Later in the survey, the pollsters learned that a majority (52 percent) did not know how an employer mandate would affect their families, and even larger majorities admitted ignorance about how a single-payer plan or individual mandate could affect them. Yet in this highly questionable exercise, Americans were asked once again to "vote" on these plans.

Even when we are not well informed, many of us still answer questions that are put to us by pollsters. Our answers can turn on a key word or phrase. Some questions tap into deep public skepticism about substantial government involvement in health care, others may reveal a belief in the importance of individual responsibility or choice, and still others may speak to our support for the goal of universal coverage. NBC News/*Wall Street Journal* pollsters attempted in March to describe the Clinton, McDermott, Chafee, Cooper, and Gramm plans (though the sponsors were not identified) and then asked whether the plans had a great deal, some, just a little, or no appeal at all. Wording that emphasized more federal involvement found little support, not surprisingly, given what we know about skepticism about federal government performance today. The poll did not reveal support or opposition to particular plans—it revealed that certain code words, phrases, or descriptions that speak to concerns about reform are going to affect responses.

Politicians and pollsters who suggest that public opinion polls provide unambiguous results about specific proposals are seriously misreading public opinion data. Democratic pollster Peter Hart was quoted during the debate as saying that the public "knows things that it hates—it knows a couple [of] things that it definitely believes—and everything else, color it confusion." Hart was right, of course.

The Fourth Wave. The fourth and final wave of polling in the 1993–1994 health care reform debate attempted to evaluate the consequences of a legislator's vote for or against a bill for that individual's chances in the November election. Such evaluations are a familiar fixture of polling today, but they are not very useful. During the debate over the North American Free Trade Agreement, for example, pollsters asked the same kind of questions. Some of the surveyors suggested that a vote for NAFTA could jeopardize a politician's chances in an election that was a year away. In fact, the issue had little impact on the campaign. Because media polls have fallen victim to the horse-race psychology that dominates political campaigns, winners and losers are regularly identified. This may make the polling exercise a little more exciting and perhaps newsworthy, but it does not tell us much about public thinking. Americans were asked by two survey organizations whether they would be likely to vote for or against a member of Congress who supported the Clinton health plan, supported other plans, or opposed major health care reform. Another organization asked, "If your member of Congress prevented any health care bill from passing Congress, would you be more likely to vote for that person, less likely, or would it not make any difference?" In the public polls, these questions are usually asked in isolation, with no points of comparison, such as a potential voter's views on other legislation, his or her perceptions of the health of the economy, or of a candidate's character. Is a voting decision ever this simple? I think not.

What We Learned from the Election

On election day, voters in California decisively defeated a single-payer initiative. In Pennsylvania, they voted against Harris Wofford, the senator who was brought to national attention in a 1991 contest in which health care figured prominently. In a Tennessee contest, they voted against Congressman Jim Cooper, a sponsor of a major alternative to President Clinton's health plan. Republicans in Congress were generally more skeptical of the administration's health care initiative than were Democrats, and it is certainly significant that not a single incumbent Republican House member or senator was defeated on election day. Nearly six in ten (58 percent) voters in the national exit poll conducted by Voter News Service (VNS) for the four networks and Associated Press said that postponing health care reform had been good "because more time is needed for discussion," while 39 percent said it was bad "because the country needs reform now." Still, more voters in House races (30 percent) told the VNS exit pollsters that health care was one of the one or two issues that "mattered most in [their] vote for Congress," more than any other issue cited. Crime was selected by 25 percent of voters; the economy and jobs, 22 percent; taxes, 18 percent; the deficit, 17 percent; Clinton's performance as president, 16 percent; time for a change, 15 percent; a candidate's experience, 11 percent; and foreign policy, 5 percent.

On the ballots they were provided at polling places, voters who participated in the exit polls were asked to check boxes that applied to them. "Currently married" was one such box. "Listen frequently to political call-in talk shows" was another. Another box asked voters to indicate that they had no health insurance. The identification was not asked in every race, but the results are interesting nonetheless. In Illinois, Michigan, Ohio, Massachusetts, and Wisconsin governors' races, about one in ten voters said they had no health insurance. In each of these races, these individuals voted for the GOP candidate. In the Florida, Maryland, Pennsylvania, Tennessee, and Texas governors' races, about the same proportion of voters indicated they had no health insurance (in Texas the percentage was slightly higher—15 percent), and they voted for the Democratic candidate. In Maine, 16 percent of voters said they had no health insurance, and a plurality of them voted for the independent candidate for governor.

Polls conducted either on election day or shortly thereafter confirm what we learned over the course of the health care debate in 1993 and 1994, and they reinforce the conclusion of profound continuity in attitudes on important dimensions of the health care issue. Once again, we found Americans expressing a high degree of satisfaction with the health care they currently receive. Concern about cost as a problem to be addressed stood out again in these surveys, as it has for many years. Americans said again that our system has problems, but they continued to be cautious about major changes that could compromise a system with many strengths. Universal coverage is a goal, but we learned again that other values are important to Americans. The support that the polls show for universal coverage exemplifies what my colleague Everett Ladd calls the "poetry of public opinion." Americans are expressing support for a general objective. They are not saying that it has to be realized immediately, nor are they providing specific directions to legislators about how to accomplish it. Nor does this goal trump other important goals of Americans. Overwhelming public support for a nuclear freeze in the early 1980s provides another example of the poetry in the polls. By their strong support in the polls for a nuclear freeze, Americans were telling Congress that reducing tensions with the Soviets was important to them. But they clearly did not want a nuclear freeze if it meant that the Soviet Union would surpass the United States in conventional or nuclear weaponry. And finally, in the health care debate and in these new polls, Americans said loudly and clearly that they were dissatisfied with federal government performance and that they had strong reservations about the effect that more federal involvement could have on our current health care system. The polls below support these points.

• Health care, as mentioned above, ranked first in the VNS exit poll of House races as one of the one or two issues that mattered most to voters. In a November 27–28, 1994, CBS News poll, more respondents cited this issue than any other as the one problem they wanted the new Congress to concentrate on first. In this same poll, about six in ten said the next Congress should try to pass health care legislation. Three in ten said it should not. The issue remains important.

• In the Public Opinion Strategies/Hamilton & Staff poll of self-identified voters conducted November 8–9, 1994, 83 percent of those surveyed said they were satisfied with their health insurance benefits and coverage. Of this group, 52 percent indicated that they were very satisfied. Ours is clearly a system with strengths. In the same poll, "health care costs [that] are too high" was cited as the most important health care problem facing the country.

• In the election night poll of voters conducted by KRC Communications Research for Robert Blendon at the Harvard University School of Public Health's Department of Health Policy and Management and the Kaiser Family Foundation, 26 percent of those surveyed said the system was in crisis, but a strong plurality (46 percent) said that "the system has major problems, but it is not in crisis." About a quarter said that the system has problems, but that none were major, and a mere 1 percent said that the system had no problems. Again, the polls showed clear recognition of a system with strengths and problems that have to be addressed.

• In the KRC poll, four in ten Americans wanted the next Congress to make modest changes in the system, a quarter wanted it left alone, and a quarter wanted a major bill enacted. (These results appear to contradict those from a survey conducted by Yankelovich Partners for *Time* and CNN on November 9 and 10. In that survey, 48 percent said that the next Congress should "make major reforms in our health care system," 29 percent said small reforms, and 19 percent said to leave the system as it is. But a more likely explanation for the different responses is that both polls show that Americans want their concerns addressed, and that depending on the wording of questions, they are pulled in the direction of answering either "major" or "modest" reforms.

The anxiety about the future that we saw in many polls in

1993 and 1994 was demonstrated again on election day. In the KRC poll, 18 percent of voters said they had grown more supportive over the past six months of Congress's enacting major health care reform. Of this group, a majority said it was because they were more worried about their family's health care than they had been six months before. Only about three in ten of this more supportive group said it was because there was more of a health care crisis.

• Both support for the goal of universal coverage and concerns about other objectives could be seen in the results of a KRC question that asked Americans whether they were willing to pay more—either in higher health insurance premiums or in higher taxes—to guarantee coverage for all Americans. A bare majority (51 percent) said they would, but nearly four in ten said they would not. Not surprisingly, Democrats and Republicans differed, with nearly seven in ten of those who voted for a Democrat on election night saying they would be willing to pay higher taxes (22 percent of this group said they would not). Of those who voted for Republican candidates, 48 percent said they would not be willing to pay more, while 43 percent said they would. A plurality (38 percent) in another question wanted Congress to guarantee health insurance coverage for all Americans, while 35 percent wanted Congress to make a start by covering some groups who do not have health insurance. Not surprisingly, children were the group that more people wanted to cover, above any other. The Public Opinion Strategies/Hamilton & Staff poll showed nearly twice as many Americans citing high costs as the most important health care problem facing the country as cited "too many Americans having no health insurance." Again, these questions show a recognition that Americans have many concerns in this area.

• The public's problems with the way the federal government is performing today were overwhelmingly evident on election day, as they had been in survey after survey during the course of this debate. Four in ten voters on the exit poll said government should do more, but 56 percent said government is doing too many things better left to business and individuals. In the KRC poll, those who had become less supportive of health care over the past six months (31 percent of the sample) gave as the primary reason that "the government wouldn't do it right." When asked in another question what worried them most about health care reform if Congress takes action, a plurality (36 percent) in the KRC poll said "there will be too much government bureaucracy." Concern about deterioration of the quality of care was cited by 22 percent, while concern about limited choice of doctors or hospitals was cited by 20 percent. In another question in the survey, Americans said private insurance companies (55 percent) and not government (24 percent) would be better at running the health insurance system. A majority (54 percent) said that state governments, not the federal government (22 percent), should take the lead in changing the health care system. In another survey conducted by Greenberg Research, Inc., for the Democratic Leadership Council on November 8 and 9, 1994, 54 percent of self-identified voters indicated that they felt disappointed with Bill Clinton as president since he took office. Of this group, nearly half said it was because he proposed big government solutions to health care reform. In the same survey, 68 percent of voters agreed with the statement, "Government always manages to mess things up."

These results suggest that the polls did not mislead the policy makers on the importance of the health care issue or on the urgency of reform. The issue is important to Americans, as it long has been. Americans want policy makers to pay attention to their concerns about it. At the same time, they are highly skeptical about more federal involvement in the health care system—particularly if that involvement compromises the parts of the system that are working well. They want reforms to be considered carefully and deliberately. They want a full discussion of the ramifications of change, not precipitous action. The weight of polling evidence today is clearly on the view of the federal government as a problem causer, not a problem solver, and Americans are not at all confident that more federal government involvement would make their (or other Americans') health care better. That is the verdict they have rendered to date.

About the Author

KARLYN H. BOWMAN is a resident fellow at the American Enterprise Institute and editor of *The American Enterprise*. From 1979 to 1989, Ms. Bowman was managing editor of *Public Opinion* magazine. She has written numerous articles on many public opinion topics, including the gender gap, foreign policy attitudes, and family issues.

Special Studies in Health Reform